YOUR KNOWLEDGE HAS VALUE

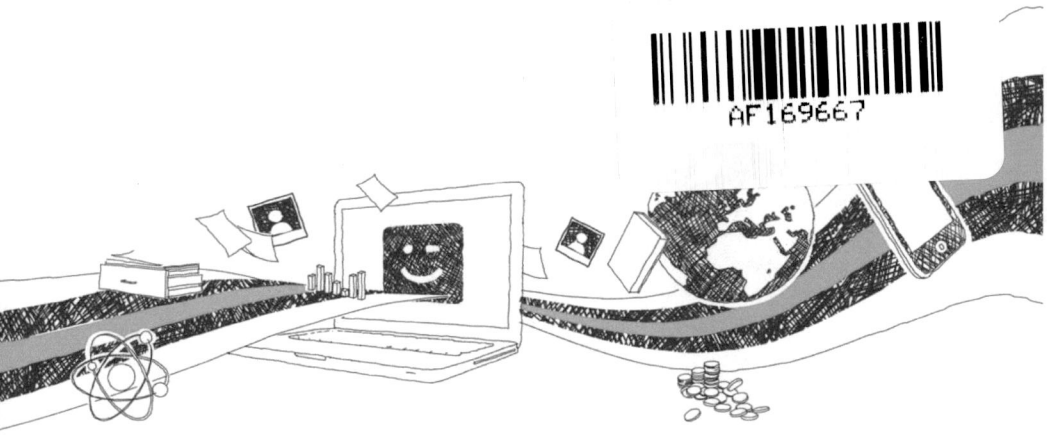

- We will publish your bachelor's and master's thesis, essays and papers

- Your own eBook and book - sold worldwide in all relevant shops

- Earn money with each sale

Upload your text at www.GRIN.com
and publish for free

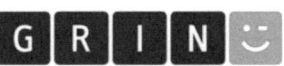

Bibliographic information published by the German National Library:

The German National Library lists this publication in the National Bibliography; detailed bibliographic data are available on the Internet at http://dnb.dnb.de .

This book is copyright material and must not be copied, reproduced, transferred, distributed, leased, licensed or publicly performed or used in any way except as specifically permitted in writing by the publishers, as allowed under the terms and conditions under which it was purchased or as strictly permitted by applicable copyright law. Any unauthorized distribution or use of this text may be a direct infringement of the author s and publisher s rights and those responsible may be liable in law accordingly.

Imprint:

Copyright © 2017 GRIN Verlag, Open Publishing GmbH
Print and binding: Books on Demand GmbH, Norderstedt Germany
ISBN: 9783668592469

This book at GRIN:

http://www.grin.com/en/e-book/381308/treatment-control-and-prevention-of-the-anthrax-disease

Patrick Kimuyu

Treatment, control and prevention of the Anthrax disease

GRIN Publishing

GRIN - Your knowledge has value

Since its foundation in 1998, GRIN has specialized in publishing academic texts by students, college teachers and other academics as e-book and printed book. The website www.grin.com is an ideal platform for presenting term papers, final papers, scientific essays, dissertations and specialist books.

Visit us on the internet:

http://www.grin.com/

http://www.facebook.com/grincom

http://www.twitter.com/grin_com

ANTHRAX

Name: Patrick K. Kimuyu

Summary

Anthrax is a bacteria-caused disease affects mammals of the bovine and caprine species, and it causes fatal deaths in humans. The most affected domestic animals include goats, sheep, cattle and horses. It is a fatal disease in animals owing to the fact that, it is transmitted from one herbivorous animal to another the same way as other zoonotic diseases. Humans acquire anthrax through three principal means: the skin, gastrointestinal tract and the respiratory tract. Anthrax toxins cause fatal effects on the central nervous system, the brain and heart. It is believed that the symptoms and signs presented in anthrax infection are as a result of the toxic effects on some vital organs and systems.

The treatment of anthrax depends on the form of anthrax involved although therapeutic agents target the disease causing pathogen, *Bacillus anthracis*. As such, antibiotics are used to destroy the anthrax causing bacteria. Some of the most potent antibiotics include penicillin, ciprofloxacin and doxycycline.

Despite the fatality associated with anthrax, reliable preventive and control measures reduce the risk of the disease. From an epidemiological perspective, prevention is usually considered as the most appropriate approach in counteracting the impacts of a given disease. Currently, anthrax is contracted through direct or indirect contact with infected animals in the endemic areas.

Anthrax toxins' toxicity is extremely fatal because it leads to sudden death if medical intervention is not availed during the initial stages of the disease infection.

Anthrax

Anthrax is a bacteria-caused disease affects mammals of the bovine and caprine species, and it causes fatal deaths in humans. The most affected domestic animals include goats, sheep, cattle and horses. It is a fatal disease in animals owing to the fact that, it is transmitted from one herbivorous animal to another, the same way as other zoonotic diseases. However, it is worth noting that anthrax disease is not common in humans (CDC 2013). Additionally, anthrax is not usually transmitted from one person to another, as it is the case in domestic and wild animals.

Humans acquire anthrax through three principal means: the skin, gastrointestinal tract and the respiratory tract. Infection through the skin is referred to as cutaneous anthrax. This form of anthrax occurs when the anthrax causing bacteria enters the body through open wounds or abrasion, primarily through making contact with the infected animal of carcass. Gastrointestinal infection occurs when an individual ingests infected beef products (CDC 2013). This is usually referred to as gastrointestinal anthrax. Respiratory or inhalation anthrax occurs when an individual inhales the anthrax bacterium spores primarily through breathing air that is contaminated with the anthrax bacteria. This occurs mostly in areas where there is anthrax outbreak. The same case may occur when humans are exposed to anthrax bacteria as a biological weapon.

Anthrax toxins cause fatal effects on the central nervous system, the brain and heart. It is believed that the symptoms and signs presented in anthrax infection are as a result of the toxic effects on some vital organs and systems. Therefore, this paper will provide an overview of anthrax disease including its pathophysiology, epidemiology, treatment, and control and prevention.

In practice, the treatment of anthrax depends on the form of anthrax involved although therapeutic agents target the disease causing pathogen, *Bacillus anthracis*. As such, antibiotics are used to destroy the anthrax causing bacteria. Some of the most potent antibiotics include penicillin, ciprofloxacin and doxycycline. These antibiotics are the most reliable treatment options for anthrax treatment, especially in humans because *Bacillus anthracis* does not exhibit resistance to beta-lactam therapeutic agents. In most cases, treatment approaches combine these antibiotics, in order to improve their potency. For instance, inhalational anthrax treatment involves a combination of ciprofloxacin as the first-line drug with another antibiotic such as penicillin. These drugs are usually administered intravenously, and they are used for 60 days to ensure that all anthrax bacteria spores are destroyed. On the other hand, cutaneous anthrax treatment involves a combination of ciprofloxacin and doxycycline, in which they are administered orally for 7 to 10 days (Vyas 2013).

Despite the fatality associated with anthrax, reliable preventive and control measures reduce the risk of the disease. From an epidemiological perspective, prevention is usually considered as the most appropriate approach in counteracting the impacts of a given disease. Currently, there are several preventive measures for anthrax. One of the most reliable preventive measures is the immunization of high risk persons with a cell-free vaccine. For instance, laboratory workers who are exposed to anthrax are advised to receive the vaccination against anthrax followed by annual boosters, in order to prevent cutaneous anthrax exposures. However, it is worth noting that, anthrax vaccine has not yet been allowed for immunization of the public. The second preventive measure is educating healthcare professionals who handle potentially infected samples on proper handling to prevent skin abrasions. Thirdly, protective clothing and proper ventilation of hazardous environments such as beef processing industries serve as appropriate measures for preventing anthrax. In addition, animal products such as hair, bone meal, wool or hides, as well as, other products of animal origin should be sterilized prior to processing. On the other hand, control of anthrax involves restricting contacts with infected animals. Animal movements, especially livestock should also be restricted to reduce transmission (State Government of Australia 2007).

Currently, anthrax is contracted through direct or indirect contact with infected animals in the endemic areas. Anthrax is common most agricultural regions such as southern and Eastern Europe, sub-Saharan Africa, Central and South-western Asia, and Central and South America. Some of the areas where anthrax is rare are Canada and the United States.

It is reported that, anthrax occurs sporadically in the endemic countries in which wild herbivores and livestock are affected. In humans, anthrax transmission has been found to occur through the use of contaminated animal products such as hides used in making drums which are imported from anthrax endemic countries (CDC 2013). In Australia, there have been outbreaks of anthrax from year-to-year, and re-emergence risks are usually high in livestock producing regions.

Anthrax disease is caused by the spore-forming Gram-positive bacterium referred to as *Bacillus anthracis* (Alibek et al. 2002). This bacterium forms resistant spores in unfavourable environment, which germinate when environmental conditions become favourable. Anthrax bacteria spores are commonly found in animal products such as wool, skins and hides. The bacterium spores survive in the soil for many decades. On the other hand, anthrax bacteria may enter into the body systems when an individual ingests beef products obtained from animals that are infected with anthrax bacteria. Anthrax bacteria may also enter into the body through skin cuts or abrasion, especially when an individual gets into direct contact with the anthrax infected beef products such as blood, milk and meat. Anthrax infection occurs more often in domestic animals than in humans. However, it is worth noting that it also affects wild animals such as elephants, hippos and buffalo.

Anthrax spores are used in warfare as a biological weapon, especially in terrorism as it was witnessed in the United States of America, in 2001, when postal mails were found to be laced with finely powdered anthrax spores.

In humans, anthrax disease manifests itself through various symptoms, which occur as a result of the anthrax toxins effects on the brain, heart and the central nervous system. *Bacillus anthracis* multiplies rapidly in the human body upon exposure. The virulence of *Bacillus anthracis* is attributed to its antiphagocytic binding proteins that are located on the bacterium's cell membrane. Upon gaining entry into the body, especially in the blood stream, it produces toxins that are responsible for the disease conditions. The most potent toxins are the lethal toxin and the oedema toxin.

In cutaneous anthrax, *Bacillus anthracis* enters the body and penetrates into the cutaneous tissue where it combines with the body's immune cells known as the macrophages. It, therefore, releases its toxins to the surrounding cutaneous tissues: thus causing oedema and brawny erythema. Thereafter, malignant pustules form within 1 to 10 days after infection. However, it is worth noting that these pustules are painless; therefore, it is difficult to suspect any microbial infection unless thorough diagnosis is conducted. The *Bacilli anthracis* are carried along the lymphatic system to the lymph nodes where they cause lymphadenopathy. This aspect leads to symptoms such as headache, fever and malaise. Myalgia, nausea and vomiting are also believed to be caused by the oedema toxin.

Infection of *Bacillus anthracis* in the oral region especially in the pharynx and the throat leads to the penetration of the bacterium into pharyngeal tissues where it releases the oedema toxin. This toxin causes necrotic ulcers and oedematous lesions on the posterior pharyngeal wall. The *Bacilli anthracis* are engulfed by the macrophages to form complexes, which are later transported along the lymphatic system to the cervical lymph nodes. *Bacillus anthracis* toxicity in the cervical lymph nodes causes enlargement of the lymph nodes and soft-tissue swellings. Oedema toxin is also believed to cause necrotic ulcers in the lymph nodes, especially in the tonsils which serve as the principal primary lymph organs in the neck region. Effects of the oedema toxin are manifested as fever, sore throat and dysphagia. Hoarseness and airway obstruction is also witnessed especially at advanced infection stages.

Gastrointestinal anthrax is believed to be asymptomatic during the initial stages of infection, but it results into severe conspicuous disease signs after lethal toxicity. *Bacillus anthracis* penetrates the gastrointestinal wall and causes intestinal tissue necrosis: thus forming ascites on the gastrointestinal wall. As a result, the patient experiences severe abdominal pain, fever and nausea. In most cases, the patient passes bloody diarrhoea due to necrosis on the intestinal wall.

Inhalation anthrax occurs when vegetative spores are trapped by macrophages on the alveolar spaces of the respiratory system. The vegetative spores acquire nourishment within the macrophages and germinate into infectious bacterium on its way to the mediastinal lymph nodes. Lethal toxin causes hemorrhagic mediastinitis, pleural effusion and pulmonary oedema leading to the production of bloody sputum. In addition, bacteria multiplication leads to bacteraemia.

Bacillus anthracis releases oedema toxin and lethal toxin, which are believed to cause toxicity in the body of the infected individual. Lethal toxin has been found to disrupt TCR signalling through inhibiting the activity of the TCR-stimulated MAP Kinase. TCR expression serves as the principal cellular activity that enhances formation of the immune response macrophages. The lethal toxin possesses a metalloprotease, which is referred to as the Lethal Factor (LF); a protective antigen that has been found to intoxicate the host cells (Ballard et al. 2009). As a result, the host's immune response to tumours and pathogens becomes impaired.

Excessive toxicity in the host's body leads to excessive production of cytokines which, in turn, causes shock and coma. Any further progression of the disease, especially when treatment interventions are not appropriate leads to a sudden death.

Anthrax toxins have been found to cause adverse effects in the brain and the central nervous system. Research studies show that lethal toxin and oedema toxin disrupts impulse transmission in the nervous system. However, there is no reliable evidence that shows how the anthrax toxins influence the central nervous system. Research reveals that the anthrax toxins inhibit the activity of Acetyl cholinesterase enzyme that is concerned with signal transmission across the synaptic cleft. Moreover, hemorrhagic reactions in the brain of an infected individual are believed to be induced by the anthrax toxins. This condition causes blockage of vital blood capillaries in the brain leading the eventual death of brain cells. Paralyses occur especially when vital brain regions are affected. On the other hand, haemolysis in the blood circulation leads to blockage of blood vessels: thus leading to cardiac failure.

Anthrax toxins' toxicity is extremely fatal because it leads to sudden death if medical intervention is not availed during the initial stages of the disease infection. Recovery of the body's immune system occurs after efficient administration of broad-spectrum antibiotics such as ciprofloxacin and doxycycline because the anthrax bacteria are either destroyed or suppressed. Consequently, TCR signalling is restored leading to the production of macrophages (Ballard et al. 2009).

Conclusively, anthrax has been observed to cause fatal health consequences in humans. It also causes mass deaths in most domestic and wild animals because; it is highly contagious. Pathogenesis of *Bacillus anthracis* is attributed to the anthrax toxins, oedema and lethal toxins. Moreover, anthrax bacterium expresses antiphagocytic proteins on its cell surface, which is believed to be the principal cause of its virulence. Its effects on the brain heart and the CNS can be attributed to its pathophysiology. Anthrax toxins cause various physiological reactions in the host's body that result into the observed disease symptoms and signs. Research shows that the anthrax toxins cause apoptosis of body cells, especially in the brain, heart and the lymph nodes, which leads to the sudden death of the infected individual (Alibek et al. 2002).

In practice, the treatment of anthrax focuses on destroying the disease causing pathogen. Therefore, antibiotics such as penicillin and other beta-lactam therapeutic agents are considered as the reliable treatment remedies.

On the other hand, prevention and control of anthrax focuses on reducing transmission through contact with infected animal carcasses because human to human transmission is rare. Some of the most reliable preventive measures include the immunization of handlers of potentially infected samples such as laboratory workers, and education on proper handling of contaminated products including animal carcasses (State Government of Victoria 2007). Currently, anthrax is endemic in agricultural regions in the world, and re-emergence risks are high in these regions.

References

Alibek, D 2002, Effect of Bacillus anthracis lethal toxin on human peripheral blood mononuclear cells, *PubMed*, vol. 527, pp. 211-5.

Ballard, J. et al. 2009, Bacillus anthracis lethal toxin disrupts TCR signalling in CD1d-restricted NKT cells leading to functional anergy. *PLoS Pathogens*, vol. 5 no.9, pp. 1-25.

CDC 2013, *Anthrax*, viewed 12 May 2017 < http://wwwnc.cdc.gov/travel/yellowbook/2014/chapter-3-infectious-diseases-related-to-travel/anthrax >

State Government of Victoria 2007, *Anthrax*, viewed 12 May 2017 < http://ideas.health.vic.gov.au/bluebook/anthrax.asp>

Vyas, J 2013, *Anthrax*, viewed 12 May 2017 < http://www.nlm.nih.gov/medlineplus/ency/article/001325.htm>

YOUR KNOWLEDGE HAS VALUE

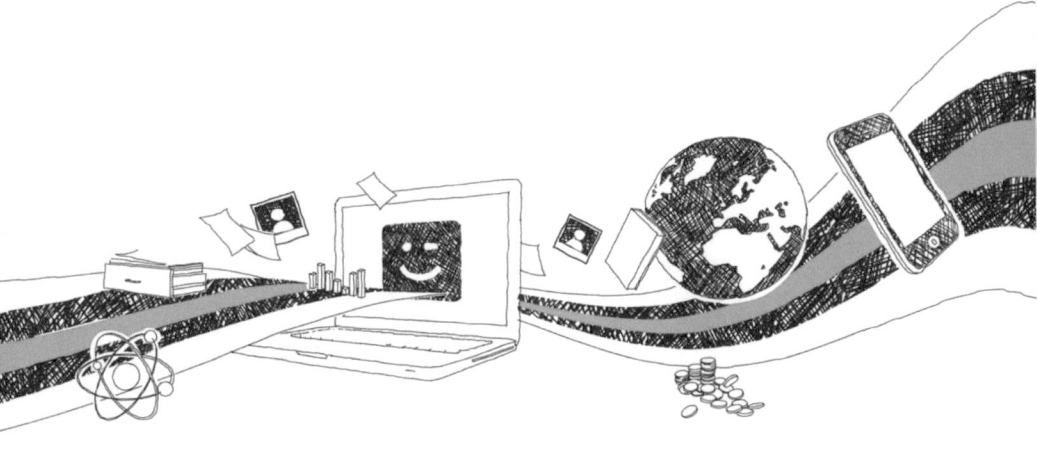

- We will publish your bachelor's and master's thesis, essays and papers

- Your own eBook and book - sold worldwide in all relevant shops

- Earn money with each sale

Upload your text at www.GRIN.com
and publish for free

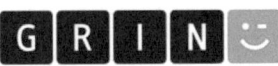